INDEX

Prologue

Within this acne based manual, you will find detailed info about this dermatological disease, which is extremely hated by young people who are getting through their puberty or by the adult ones who have this condition as a chronic one. Besides, it offers recommendations and advice on how you can treat it.

It is highly important getting to know the problem´s root so you can be able to fight it, that's why I'm inviting you to read this book based on the author's experience, where it teaches you all the things you need to know about the acne, which is very common nowadays and it causes low self-esteem and insecurity.

May it be helpful.

Dr. Rosmely Leonardo Cuas

Acne Treaty/ Adult Acne
Introduction

From my perspective, this is not a book, but rather a practical and straightforward manual that I wrote intending to help people overcome that unpleasant situation that arises when they get those annoying pimples on their face.

Some people are genetically programmed never to get acne in their lives.

This handbook is for us who have such a genetic deficiency. However, it is designed to treat this problem in the most natural way possible understanding that our body's natural balance is perfect health.

One of the laws of nature that can be most generally applied to almost all (if not all) areas of life is the Universal Law of Cause and Effect. This simple law states that every effect has its cause, and every cause has its effect.

As in almost everything, issues in the relationship between an individual and its physical body can cause diseases.

You are a being, not a body. Your body is one thing. When the relationship you have with your body is less than harmonious, there is always the possibility to result in disease. Once you find out where the cause of a problem is, you can eliminate that cause, and by doing so automatically, the problem disappears.

The subject that concerns us today is acne; when we discover its cause, we will automatically eliminate it. That's what this book is about.

The author is not a doctor or specialist. The author is a simple researcher, a curious mind, a thinker, and an analytical observer. The advice given in this book is the result of personal research and self-experimentation in that area.

Part One

What is the skin?

The skin is the coat of cells and proteins that covers all the physical constitutions that form your body. It is the largest organ in the body. Skin is like a radiator; it helps us maintain the perfect body temperature all the time; it is the window of physical sensations to our brain, pleasant or unpleasant, with it we feel.

Hundreds of thousands of bacteria live on every square inch of our skin. Over 500,000 particles are shed from our dead skin every hour.

The skin builds itself, and every month or so we have a new skin.

What is acne?

Technical description:

Acne is a pathology, inflammatory, and infectious cutaneous (of the skin), that involves the hair follicles and the sebaceous glands.
Acne has inflammatory lesions, cysts, and pimples that spread over the face, back, and chest.

When a person suffers from acne, bumps grow on its face, back, and chest; these usually differ in size and shape depending on the particular case sustained by the individual. The sebaceous glands of the face are connected to the nervous system. If the nervous system is overstimulated, these glands will produce more sebum than usual, creating the right conditions for acne development.

Adult Acne

This affects more than 30% of women over 25 years and 7% of men and is called "hormonal acne".

Some of the differences between this and acne vulgaris is that most of the lesions are inflammatory and deep.

Psychological effects of acne:

The reason for this section is to let the reader know that the author understands in his flesh his suffering.

I have suffered from this disgusting and unpleasant disease for years.
The thoughts that come into the minds of some people who suffer from acne are negative and counterproductive.
When those episodes of acne breakouts would come, I would lose heart; I didn't want to go to work, I felt embarrassed, it's like you think that others think that having acne is wrong with you. You know it's not your fault, but you're supposed to do something about it , what many people don't know that maybe you've done everything you can do and yet the problem is not solved.

I lost interest in going to the gym, contact with humans with healthy skin became uncomfortable.

I didn't go to parties or social events of any kind. When you have acne, it's like life stops. The only thing you think about is waiting for time to pass to see if it eventually disappears. Luckily this is not normal (or at least it shouldn't be).

But, which is the cause?

Your face is a mirror of what's going on inside you! Your body is a perfect machine. That has computer-like programming.
This programming is found in the reservoirs that scientists call "Genes." It is in the genes where all the natural mechanisms of the body are found.
The body is naturally programmed for several vital biological functions; ah here we are interested in its EXCRETION or ELIMINATING.

Eliminate what?

To eliminate toxins that enter your body in the form of food. These toxins are what are producing your acne. This is the secret cause of those bumps on your face, back, and chest. Your body has a system of eliminating toxins, perhaps the most perfect system in existence, but when this system is corrupted in some way, your body has no choice but to get rid of the contaminants through, if that's it; SKIN! That is why acne exists; it is nothing more or less than your body trying to release toxins that your liver, small intestine, and other organs have not been able to eliminate because of the overload of aggressive foods.

Part Two

Let's understand some issues first:

What is the lymphatic system?

The lymphatic system is a channel that carries fluid called lymph.
Lymph contributes to the cleaning of tissues and the elimination of waste, toxins, and pathogenic microorganisms.

This system is made up of lymph channels that are a network of vessels, much like blood vessels that cover all the tissues of the body. All the fluids, salts, and proteins filtered by this system end up in the bloodstream. In this way, this system carries the toxins to the skin, causing the irritations and infections characteristic of acne.

Metabolism.

Metabolism is the set of physical and biochemical processes that take place in every cell of our body.

It is all the process that takes place in the body to transform food into energy for the body's natural functioning. It transforms food into its molecular form, converts it into glucose, and that glucose feeds the cells that turn it into energy.

It is dynamic, continuous, and autonomous. Metabolism is involved in everything that happens in your body, such as brain function, enzymes, immune system, digestion, growth, nutrient absorption, hormonal regulation, and a lot more.

There are certain factors that affect your metabolism: these are the main ones. Food and Exercise.

Endocrine System.

It is formed by the group of endocrine glands, which produce and release the hormones that travel through the bloodstream. Hormones perform a similar function to neurotransmitters; they transmit messages. The number of functions that are intimately related to hormones is impressive, among them hunger, thirst, sexual behavior, fighting, aggression, etc.

However, the relationship between the nervous and endocrine systems is close. The hormone that concerns us most is called "androgens" since this is the leading cause of hormonal acne. With the increase of this hormone, the skin's sebaceous glands are stimulated, causing them to produce more sebum than usual and thus obstructing the follicle, creating the right conditions for the acne bacteria to infect the skin. Stress is a cause of late acne; it increases the levels of cortisol and androgenic hormones, increasing the sebum and skin fat.

Keep in mind that acne and stress can create a
vicious circle where both feed off each other:
you get stressed out, and you get acne = you
get acne, and you get stressed out.
The nervous system (passive and active)
The nervous system is divided into two parts:
sympathetic and parasympathetic (active and
passive).
It processes all the stimuli the body receives
to create a reaction.

In conjunction with the endocrine system, the
nervous system regulates and coordinates all
functions of the body.
There are two types of nervous systems; these
are passive and the active:
In some people, a passive nervous system is
dominant, while in others, an active nervous
system is dominant.

Acne is characteristic of people with a dominant
excited, nervous system.
This is because this type of nervous system is
easily out of control with the diet; when fat is
consumed, it will produce unbalanced immune
and hormonal systems, and when the body's
natural defense is deficient, the natural hormonal
production, causes acne infections.

Some of the foods that overstimulate the active nervous systems are: Salt
Chocolate Saturated fats Sugar

Part Three

You **a** re the Cause

I claim that you are the cause of your acne because it is simply caused by feeding, and you are feeding yourself.
Contrary to what dermatologists and scientific studies say that acne is not caused by what you eat because this logic would be this way: you eat fat, then the fat comes out of your face forming the acne outbreaks.

This is not the way that feeding is causing your acne. Still, by feeding yourself incorrectly, you are getting your metabolism and nervous system out of control. As a result, your endocrine system does too, (that is why these body systems were mentioned earlier).

It causes hormonal acne and stimulates androgens to produce more male hormones than necessary. In turn, this causes the excessive production of sebum in the face and the lowering of the immune system, causing bacteria to thrive on your skin and produce those nasty skin infections.

A different point of view, a paradigm shift. From now on, we will have a different viewpoint regarding acne and all diseases.

From now on, we will see acne as the result of inappropriate behavior; that is, we will see acne as the product of unhealthy eating, lack of rest, anxiety, and stress rather than as a disease in itself. For this reason, we will always treat the cause but not the symptom.

When we see acne on our skin or someone else's, we will know that it can be eliminated from the root by uncovering the body's natural detoxification system. Once this system is detoxified, the skin will return to NORMAL.

Dermatology

Dermatologists say, (and I have been told this personally), and I remember hearing it in a documentary: that according to scientific studies, acne is never a product of food, yet millions of people claim that our acne worsens after eating certain foods in particular.
I remember that for a while I lived in Long Island, NY, in front of my house there was a trendy pizza restaurant in that neighborhood, a friend who saw my acne problem (and who had clean skin) told me that every time he ate pizza from that place, he would get at least a pimple on his face.

I love chocolate, but I have to abstain from eating it frequently because it's almost automatic that I get pimples after eating it. That's why we mentioned earlier that your body is unique and reacts uniquely to certain foods. It seems that chocolate is a stimulant of the nervous system and the androgen glands that cause a sudden rise in androgen production and turns sebum on the skin of the face. As a result, then the immune system drops, and the acne as bacteria thrives.

Treatment

There are multiple medications for acné treatment. However, nobody ever guarantees that it will be the definitive cure; what dermatologists tell you is that acne can simply disappear one day and not come back anymore.

There are some of those medications that are effective such as isotretinoin. This medicine is effective, but only the first time it is taken. I took it and cleaned my face for a whole year after taking it for two months.

This medicine does dry out your skin to a point where bacteria cannot thrive. It also makes your eyes and lips extra dry until your lips break dry.
 It is also harmful to the liver, it should be taken with a lot of water, and while drinking

it, you should drink more water than usual to
avoid damaging your liver.
It can also produce brain pressure and brain
tumors. (According to doctors).

As you can see, modern medicine is deficient
regarding finding a cure for acne and has only
succeeded in producing treatments that can
make you sicker. Besides, it seems that their
goal is only to sell you a treatment forever.
There are also lots of soaps and creams that,
in the long run, many of them end up
damaging your skin. I recommend finding a
cleanser that doesn't harm your skin too much
so that you can wash your face in the
morning, in the afternoon, and at night, that's
enough.
We who are genetically prone to acne should
help the skin a little with some pure soap and
a natural mask from time to time.

I recommend making tomato masks; it kills
bacteria and leaves the skin very soft and
natural.

Part Four

The Solution

The solution to this condition becomes almost apparent at this point. The reader will have deduced that sick skin is nothing more or less than deficient nutrition. Therefore, the definitive solution is a healthy, clean diet. Without giving too much thought to the matter, I recommend that the reader start designing a proper eating plan in which his body naturally cleanses itself.

Within 28 to 60 days or so you will be able to see the positive changes in your skin, I also recommend helping your body with natural dietary supplements such as intestinal cleansing tablets and live enzymes to restore your intestinal flora and also perform a liver cleanse with natural pills such as:

Liver Cleanse: Detoxifier and Regenerator
Digestive Enzyme
Colon Cleanse.

Ask a nutritionist how often you should take
these supplements. The purpose is internal
cleansing; this is something simple. Just tell
him you want to cleanse your colon,
intestines, and liver.

Diet and nutrition

Creating healthy eating habits not only helps
your health and guarantees a longer and
healthier life but is also characteristic of
organized and self-respecting people.
Eating is a very personal thing; everyone eats
differently. However, certain fundamental
dietary principles can be applied to help clear
up acne naturally.

Eat fruit in the morning at least five times a
week, if not every day. Fruit helps your
digestive system, and your intestines perform

the natural detoxification process of the body more effectively.

Drink water; fall in love with water, water is medicinal, remember that your body is composed of 70% water. Drink a glass of water on an empty stomach, make this a daily routine, after a short time your body will get used to the point that the first thing you will feel in the morning when you wake up will be thirst. I do this every day. It will get your organs working.

Don't eat red meat more than twice a week; it costs your body more work to digest, try to eat white meat and fish, or anything else you like to eat.

Exercise:

Have you ever seen an athlete with skin problems? Or with a health problem in general? Isn't it very rare?

The reason is the many benefits to the human body from regular exercise. Exercise for 30 to 40 minutes a day at least four days a week. Besides balancing your hormone production, which is already very positive for your health, it contributes to our overall health.

 It increases your production of endorphins, which is the happiness hormone. You will feel better, increase your energy levels, sleep better, etc.

Exercise speeds up your metabolism, reduces stress, balances your nervous system and endocrine system, improves your quality of life, increases your attractiveness, distracts you, and increases your self-esteem and detoxifies your body.

Natural Products Recommendations:

In this section, you will find the recommended products I have personally used, which will help you detoxify your body.

Remember that this manual's fundamental principle is "Body detoxification", since it is the main reason for acne.
Something to take into account is that with a detox, you will also see other advantages that only you will perceive since internal cleansing is always positive for our health in general.

Face cleanser:

As mentioned before, people with genetic deficiencies and therefore are acne-prone should always wash their faces with a different soap than the one used for bathing.
 Let there be no doubt about this: our face and places affected by acne are more delicate than other parts of the body.
Therefore, a soap with a small percentage of salicylic acid will be effective when combined with the other products I recommend.
The soap I use is:

Asepxia

It contains 2% salic acid, used to treat various skin conditions.

Use the soap in the morning and before you go to sleep (if you can wash your face in the afternoon, that's better too, so you can do it three times a day).

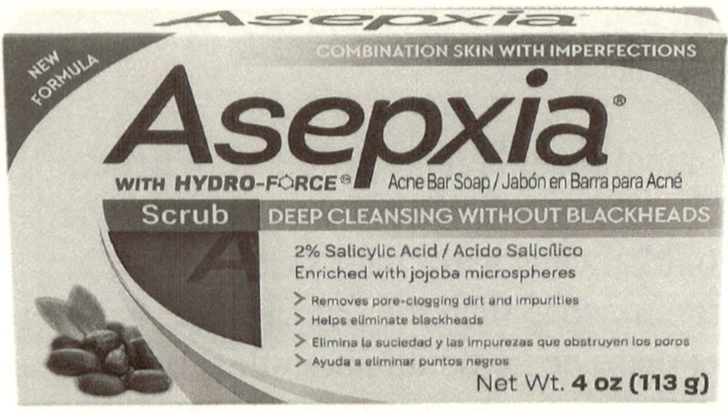

Colon Cleanse

Colon Cleanse is a natural product made from herbs; it comes in the form of oral capsules (take them with plenty of water).
The suggested use is as follows:

Take two pills before you go to sleep, and that's it.
The next day you will feel like going to the bathroom with a little more drive than usual.
This is natural since the capsules take effect at night while you sleep.
You'll probably go to the bathroom two or three times in the morning.
Try to take it on days you're home, like days off.
It is advisable to do this for three days in a row, if possible.
I do it at least once a month, even if it's once because I take better care of what I eat and clean my body more often.

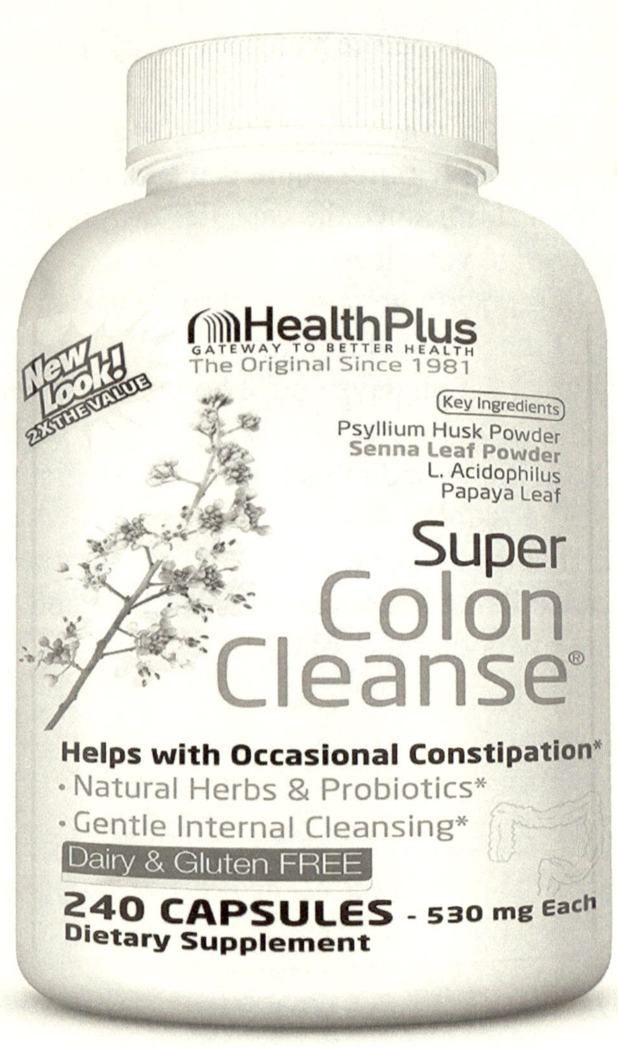

Liver Cleanse:

The liver is a vital organ. Its function is magnificent; it is a filter that removes and eliminates unwanted toxins that enter into your body through food, air, and even by skin absorption.

Its job is to remove toxins, but it can get a little clogged up from time to time, so we know how to clean it up.

Just by cleaning our liver, our health will generally improve, and our skin will be healthier.

These also come in capsules, and its suggested use is as follows:

Take two capsules, 20 to 30 minutes before lunch with plenty of water.

You should do this until you finish the 60 capsules in the bottle. That would be 30 days—a whole month.

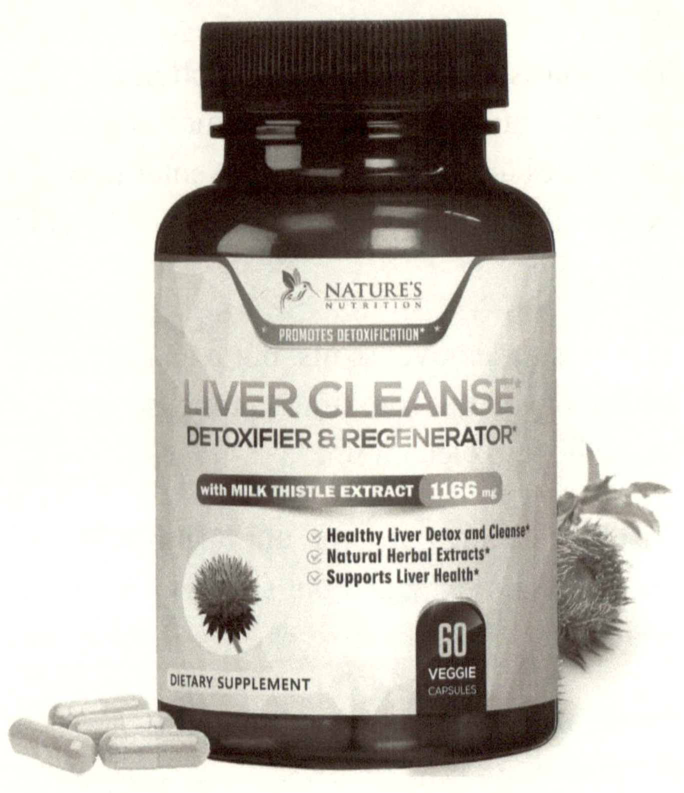

Turmeric:

Turmeric is a medicinal plant with an elongated yellowish root.
It is a condiment used in many places in the world.
It has fascinating medicinal properties, among them:

Its anti-inflammatory, antioxidant,
antibacterial, and digestive action. Therefore,
it provides several benefits for your health,
such as
Regulates the intestinal flora (vital)
Detoxifies the liver (vital)
Stimulates the immune system (which in turn
fights acne bacteria)
Improves blood circulation
Helps in weight loss
Improves digestion
All this, among other interesting things. Do
some research about its benefits, and you'll
see.
Its suggested use is as follows:
Take three capsules daily, one in the morning,
one in the afternoon and one in the evening.

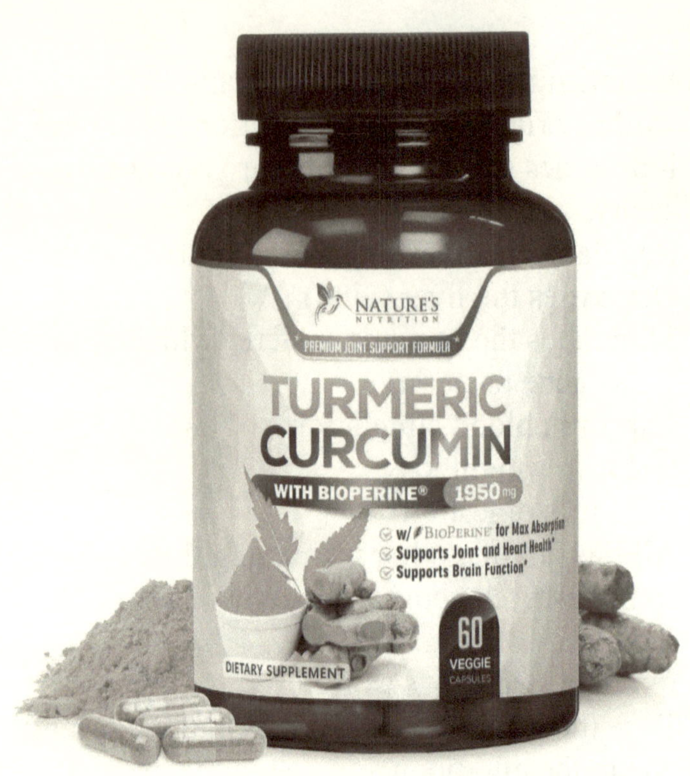

NATURE'S
NUTRITION
PREMIUM JOINT SUPPORT FORMULA
TURMERIC
CURCUMIN
WITH BIOPERINE®   1950 mg
w/ BioPerine® for Max Absorption
Supports Joint and Heart Health*
Supports Brain Function*
60 VEGGIE CAPSULES
DIETARY SUPPLEMENT

Digestive enzymes:

Digestive enzymes will be of great help in improving your metabolism and digestive processes.

It will also help you detoxify your bowel.

Its suggested use is as follows:

You can take 1 to 3 capsules a day after a meal.

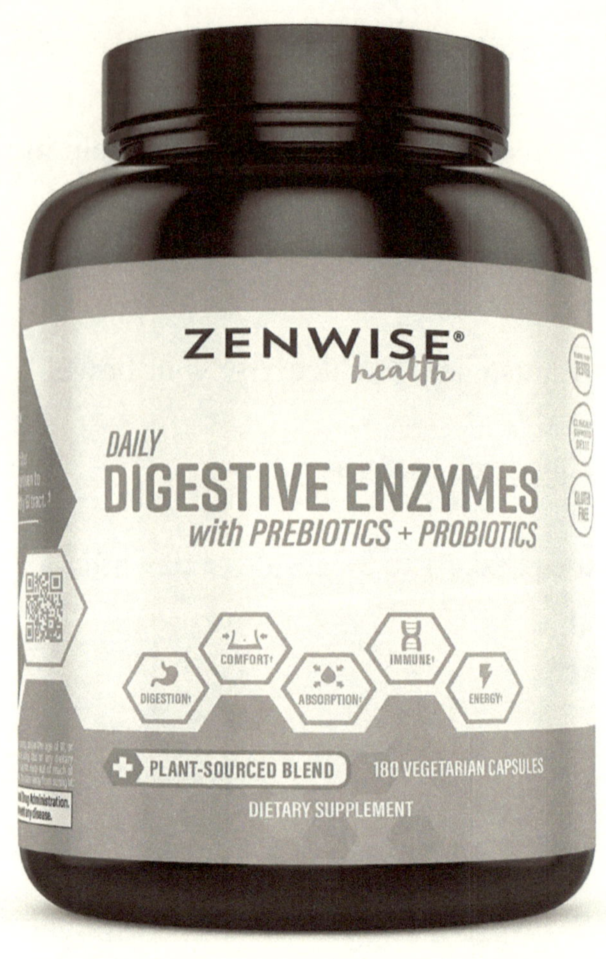

A New Skin

As you may have noticed, skin health is simply the result of a particular lifestyle, a lifestyle that leads to healthier skin. New skin will result from applying the simple tips given in this handbook.

Remember that your skin regenerates itself daily, but it takes between 28 and 60 days for your body to reproduce 100% of your skin cells. This means that every 28 days or so, we have new skin. Every change in your diet and lifestyle will be reflected in your skin condition, and this will be at least 28 days after you have started with this change.

To a new skin, I wish you lots of health!

Appreciation

I want to sincerely thank you reader for taking the time to read this humble little work. I hope the information in this book has been helpful and has added value to your life.

Special thanks to Dr. Rosmely Leonardo for reviewing my work and giving it the go-ahead.

Thanks to my friend Dawn Spaw for reviewing the English version.

Thanks to my family and friends for taking the time to review it too, to Catherine, Andy, Minelli and my mother!

Thank you so much!